Summaries for Undergraduate Medical Students

REDHWAN AL-NAGGAR

MUHAMED OSMAN

MAHFOUDH ABDULGHANI

ISBN: 1492208205
ISBN-13:978-1492208204

DEDICATION

This book is dedicated to our medical students who have been a source of continuous stimulation.

Redhwan, Osman and Mahfoudh

CONTENTS

PREFACE

The aim of this work is to assist undergraduate medical students in academic excellence. This book is based on experience of the expertise in their areas, and based on practical experiences of the authors in academic teaching and assessing students' performance.

The book gives practical MCQs with short answers for the wrong answers to help students understand different subjects. Here are concise and comprehensive MCQs with short answers in Public Health, Pathology and Pharmacology. While this book aimed for undergraduate students, it is a helpful resource for beginning academics and health professionals.

Redhwan Ahmed Al-Naggar; Ph.D (Community Medicine) Consultant Preventive Medicine, Faculty of Medicine, Universiti Teknologi MARA Malaysia.

Muhamed T. Osman; M.B.Ch.B., M.Sc., Ph.D (Pathology); Consultant Pathologist, Faculty of Medicine, Universiti Teknologi MARA Malaysia.

Mahfoudh Abdulghani; Ph.D (Pharmacology) Consultant Pharmacologist, International Medical School, Management and Science University, Malaysia

1 PUBLIC HEALTH

1.1 Questions without Answers

1. Risk factors of hypertension

   A. Excess salt intake.

   B. Overweight.

   C. Prolong extreme stress.

   D. Potassium deficiency.

   E. Physical activity.

2. The cancer that is not the commonest occupational cancer

   A. Lung cancer.

   B. Bladder cancer.

   C. Leukaemia.

   D. Skin cancer.

   E. Breast cancer.

3. The advantage of dietary fiber intake on health

   A. Reduces the tendency to constipation.

   B. Reduced incidence of coronary heart disease.

C. Reduces the post-prandial glucose levels in the blood.

D. Reduces risk for developing diabetes.

E. Increases risk for developing obesity.

4. The water soluble vitamins

A. Vitamin C.

B. Vitamin B-Complex.

C. Biotin.

D. Vitamin D.

E. Vitamin E.

5. The example of distress

A Getting married.

B Getting a new job.

C Getting breast cancer.

D Death of relatives.

E Having an examination.

6. The mental symptom of stress

A Distraction

B Confusion.

C Nail biting.

D Sweating.

E Fainting.

7. WHO definition of health includes

A Spiritual well-being.

B Physical well-being.

C Social well-being.

D Mental well-being.

E Occupational well-being.

8. The risk factors within a person's control

A Age.

B Family history.

C Weight.

D Gender.

E Race.

9. Regarding warning sign of cancer

A A sore that does not heal.

B Unusual bleeding or discharge.

C Change in bowel or bladder habits.

D Nagging cough or hoarseness.

E Indigestion or difficulty swallowing.

10. The example of primary prevention

A Breast-self examination

B Vitamin A supplementation

C Polio immunization

D Ioniazid (INH) to a baby breastfed by a sputum positive tubercular mother

E Pap smear test

11. The avoidable stress

A Road rage.

B Family problems.

C Computer burnout.

D Hurrying up

E Watching the news.

12.The personal prevention measures from Dengue fever

A Gambusia fish.

B Solid waste management.

C Clothing to reduce exposed skin.

D Space spraying

E Applied replants on the exposure skin.

13. Diseases associated with obesity

A Cardiovascular diseases

B Diabetes mellitus type 2

C Sleep apnea

D Dengue

E H1N1

14. The medication that can be given to the Dengue patients

A Aspirin

B Paracetamol

C Tetracycline

D Amoxicillin

E Ciprofloxacin

15. The types of scientific research articles

A Review articles.

B Meta analysis.

C Original articles.

D Magazine articles.

E Newspaper articles.

16. Institutional ethics committee should

A include professionals.

B include community representatives.

C not include lawyers.

D include researchers.

E include statisticians.

17. In a community, an increase in new cases of HIV will

A Increase incidence rate

B Increase prevalence rate

C Increase morbidity rate

D Increase mortality rate

E Decrease incidence rate

18. Regarding risk groups of Malaria

A Pregnant women

B Travelers

C Refugees

D Aboriginal people

E Armed personal

19. The following is a fundamental medical science that focuses on the distribution and determinants of disease frequency in human population

A Biology.

B Public health.

C Bio-statistics.

D Epidemiology.

E Statistic.

20. The purpose of a double blind study

A Avoid subject bias.

B Avoid observer bias and sampling variation

C Avoid observer bias.

D Avoid subject bias and doesn't matter for observer.

E Guard against both experimenter bias and placebo effects.

21. The following vitamin is lost during rice polishing

A Carotene

B Thiamine

C Cyanocobalamin

D Ascorbic Acid

E Vitamin E

22. Double blind study

A Participant is only not aware of the group allocation and treatment received.

B Neither the participant nor the researcher is aware of the group allocation and treatment received.

C Participant and investigator are aware of the group allocation and treatment received.

D Researcher is only not aware of the group allocation and treatment received.

E Participant is only aware of the group allocation and treatment received.

23. Regarding cross-sectional study:

A Follow up is not a necessary feature.

B Cause and effect relationship can be established

C All cases are seen at one point in time.

D More useful for chronic diseases.

E describes what exists at time of study

24. Regarding the ideal target population in Measles control in emergency situation

A Routine vaccination.

B 14 years and above.

C 5 years of age.

D 14 years and below

E 10 years and above

25. Health education may often fail due to communication barriers between the educator and community. Which of the following is the main communication barrier?

A Physiological.

B Psychological.

C Environmental.

D Physiological but not Psychological

E Psychological but not Environmental.

26. To call a person a drug addict, which of the following criteria must be satisfied?

A Psychological dependence.

B Physical dependence.

C Development of tolerance

D Psychological or physical dependence

E Dependent on an addictive substance

27. Fat content is highest in:

A Chicken drumstick

B Chicken breast

C Beef

D Salmon

E Tuna

28. Macronutrient includes

A Proteins

B Fats

C Carbohydrates

D Iron

E Zinc

29. Vitamins are a class of

A Inorganic compounds.

B Organic compounds.

C Either Organic or inorganic compounds

D Neither organic nor inorganic compounds

E Organic and inorganic compounds

30. 'A clinically manifest disease of man resulting from an infection' is called:

A Infectious disease.

B Contagious disease.

C Iatrogenic disease.

D Nosocomial disease.

E Communicable disease

31. 'Number of deaths due to a particular cause (or in a specific age group) per 100 (or 1000) total deaths' is known as:

A Prevalence rate

B Proportional mortality rate

C Case fatality rate

D Standardized mortality rate

E Incidence rate

32. A study was conducted in Malaysia with a group of 200 breast cancer patients to determine the quality of life in a single institute. The design of this study is:

A Case control study

B Retrospective cohort study

C Concurrent cohort study

D Cross sectional study

E Descriptive study

33. Highest vitamin A content is seen in:

A Lemon

B Apple

C Tomato

D Spinach

E Broccoli

34. Study of time, place and person distribution of health related events is known as:

A Descriptive epidemiology

B Experimental epidemiology

C Analytical epidemiology

D Clinical epidemiology

E Epidemiology

35. If the drug prevent mortality but does not affect cure, then which of the following will be true:

A Incidence will decrease

B Incidence will increase

C Prevalence will decrease

D Prevalence will increase

E Incidence and prevalence will increase

36. What most describes an abstract of scientific research article

A The most read section

B A one-two page summary of the research.

C Should contain information on minor content of the study.

D Not contain the key words of the research.

E Should include the objective of the study

37. Prevalence of a disease

A Can only be determined by a cohort study.

B Is the number of new cases in a defined population

C Describes the balance between incidence, mortality and recovery

D Is the best measure of disease frequency in etiological studies

E Can determine by cross-sectional study.

38. Vigorous physical activity is bicycling

A 9 miles per hour.

B more than 10 miles per hour.

C less than 10 miles per hour.

D less than 15 Kilometer per hour.

E more than 15 Kilometer per hour.

39. The proximate principles food

A Proteins.

B Fats.

C Carbohydrates.

D Vitamins.

E Minerals.

40. Assessment methods of nutritional status include

A Clinical methods

B Anthropometric methods

C Biochemical methods.

D Laboratory Methods

E Dietary evaluation methods

41. The following is a body building food

A Grilled chicken

B Boiled egg

C Peanut butter

D Brown rice

E Cheese

42. The daily fat requirement should be ________ of total daily energy intake?

A 10%

B 15%

C 20%

D 30%

E 40%

43. The following is unsaturated fat

A Wheat

B Sunflower

C Olive

D Corn

E Butter

44. The following is essential amino acids

A Lysine

B Alanine

C Tryptophan

D Phenylalanine

E Leucine

45. Diana is 22 years old, eats and then vomits secretly, What eating disorder does she suffer from?

A Compulsive overeating

B Anorexia nervosa

C Bulimia nervosa

D Binge eating disorder

E Body dysmorphic disorder

46. 'Keeping the frequency of illness within acceptable limits' is best described as

A Elimination

B Eradication

C Control

D Surveillance

E Observation

47. What technique of weight assessment is based on the relationship of weight to height?

A Body consumption index

B Body mass index

C Hydrostatic weight

D Waist to hip ratio

E Skinfold caliper test

48. The presence of an infectious agent on a body surface and/or surgical instruments and dressings is known as

A Infection

B Infestation

C Contamination

D Pollution

E Contagion

49. Regarding information in the international death certificate

A The certificate deals with the immediate and also the underlying cause

B The certificate deals with the immediate cause only

C The certificate deals with the underlying cause only

D Other morbid conditions not related to the cause of death are not included

E The certificate should include the bio-data

50. The food that is not accepted as a reference protein:

A Human milk

B Cow's milk

C Hen's egg

D Soybean

E Goat milk

1.2 Questions with Answers

1. Risk factors of hypertension

T A. Excess salt intake.

T B. Overweight.

T C. Prolong extreme stress.

T D. Potassium deficiency.

F E. Physical activity because physical activity and regular exercise can protect against hypertension. The WHO recommends at least 30 minutes of regular, moderate-intensity physical activity on most days of the week to reduce the risk of diseases.

2. The cancer that is not the commonest occupational cancer is

T A. Lung cancer

T B. Bladder cancer

T C. Leukaemia

F D. Skin cancer because Employees who work outdoors for all or part of the day are at risk of skin cancer. This is because solar radiation is carcinogenic to humans1. All skin types can be damaged by exposure to solar ultraviolet radiation (UVR). Damage is permanent and irreversible and increases with each exposure. The main cause is excessive exposure to the sun's harmful ultra violet (UV) radiation.

T E. Breast cancer

3. The advantage of dietary fiber intake on health

T A. Reduces the tendency to constipation

T B. Associated with reduced incidence of coronary heart disease

T C. Reduces the post-prandial glucose levels in the blood

T D. Reduces risk for developing diabetes

F E. Increases risk for developing obesity because Dietary fiber intake provides many health benefits. A generous intake of dietary fiber reduces risk for developing coronary heart disease, stroke, hypertension, diabetes and obesity. Furthermore, increased consumption of dietary fiber improves serum lipid concentrations, lowers blood pressure, improves blood glucose control in diabetes, promotes regularity, aids in weight loss, and appears to improve immune function.

4. The water soluble vitamins

T A. Vitamin C.

T B. Vitamin B-Complex.

T C. Biotin.

F D. Vitamin D. becausevitamin D is a group of fat-soluble vitamin responsible for intestinal absorption of calcium and phosphate. The body can synthesize vitamin D when sun exposure is adequate.

F E. Vitamin E. because vitamin E is a major lipid-soluble antioxidant, which protects lipoproteins and the unsaturated fatty acids in cell membranes. Fighting against the effects of free radicals derived from oxygen and environmental pollutants, vitamin E reduces the rate of free radical attack on the polyunsaturated fatty acids in membrane phospholipids and at other biologically important sites.

5. The example of distress

A F Marriage because Marriage can cause eustress which is the positive cognitive response to stress that is healthy, or gives one a feeling of fulfillment or other positive feelings. Eustress refers to a positive response one has to a stressor, which can depend on one's current feelings of control, desirability, location, and timing of the stressor. Eustress has also been positively correlated with life satisfaction and well-being.

B F Getting a new job because Getting a new job can cause eustress

C T Getting breast cancer.

D T Death.

E F Examination because Examination can cause eustress

6. The mental symptom of stress

A T Lack of concentration.

B T Confusion.

C T Nail biting.

D F Sweating because Sweating is a physical symptom of the stress

E F Fainting because Fainting is a physical symptom of the stress

7. WHO definition of health includes

A F Spiritual well-being because Spiritual well-being is not included in the WHO definition because it is defined as "Health is a state of complete physical, mental and social well-being and not merely the absence of disease or infirmity.

B T Physical well-being

C T Social well-being

D T Mental well-being

E F Occupational well-being because occupational well-being is also not included in WHO definition

8. The risk factors within a person's control

A T Age.

B T Family history.

C F Weight because weight is a risk factor that can be modified by healthy life-style such as regular exercise and physical activities

D T Gender.

E T Race.

9. Regarding warning sign of cancer

A T A sore that does not heal

B T Unusual bleeding or discharge

C T Change in bowel or bladder habits

D T Nagging cough or hoarseness

E T Indigestion or difficulty swallowing

10. The example of primary prevention

A F Breast-self examination because Breast-self examination is a secondary prevention for breast cancer

B T Vitamin A supplementation

C T Polio immunization

D T Ioniazid (INH) to a baby breastfed by a sputum positive tubercular mother

E F Pap smear test because Pap smear is considered a secondary prevention measures against cervical cancer

11. The avoidable stress

A F Road rage because Road rage is classified as unavoidable stress due to the civilization and rapid development of the world.

B F Family problems because family stress is also classified as unavoidable stress because all family members will be affected by family problem directly or indirectly.

C F Computer burnout because computer burnout is considered unavoidable stress due to the civilization and rapid development of the world.

D T Hurrying

E T Watching the news.

12. The personal prevention measures from Dengue fever

A F Gambusia fish because Gamusia fish Is a biological prevention methods

B F Solid waste management because solid waste management is environment prevention

C T Clothing to reduce exposed skin.

D F Space spraying because space spraying is considered as environmental prevention not a personal prevention

E T Applied replants on the exposure skin.

13. Diseases associated with obesity

A T Cardiovascular diseases

B T Diabetes mellitus type 2

C T Sleep apnea

D F Dengue because No association between obesity and Dengue

E F H1N1 because No association between obesity and H1N1

14. The medication that can be given to the Dengue patients

A F Aspirin because Aspirin and non-steroidal anti-inflammatory drugs should be avoided as these drugs may worsen the bleeding tendency associated with some of these infections.

B T Paracetamol

C T Tetracycline

D T Amoxicillin

E T Ciprofloxacin

15. The types of scientific research articles

A T Review articles.

B T Meta analysis.

C T Original articles.

D F Magazine articles because An article in the magazine is not considered a scientific research article because it does not follow the scientific research methods.

E F Newspaper articles because An article in the magazine is not considered a scientific research article because it does not follow the scientific research methods.

16. Institutional ethics committee should

A T include professionals.

B T include community representatives.

C F not include lawyers because The research committee should include lawyers in order to advice in terms of human rights.

D T include researchers.

E T include statisticians.

17. In a community, an increase in new cases of HIV will

A T Increase incidence rate

B F Increase prevalence rate because Increase in new cases of HIV will increase the incidence rate not the prevalence rate.

C F Increase morbidity rate because Increase in new cases of HIV will increase the incidence rate not the morbidity rate.

D F Increase mortality rate because Increase in new cases of HIV will increase the incidence rate not the mortality rate.

E F Decrease incidence rate because Increase in new cases of HIV will increase the incidence rate not decrease in incidence rare.

18. Regarding risk groups of Malaysia

A T Pregnant women

B T Travelers

C T Refugees

D T Aboriginal people

E T Armed personal

19. The following is a fundamental medical science that focuses on the distribution and determinants of disease frequency in human population

A F Biology because Biology is a natural science concerned with the study of life and living organisms, including their structure, function, growth, evolution, distribution, and taxonomy.

B F Public health because Public health is "the science and art of preventing disease, prolonging life and promoting health through the organized efforts and informed choices of society, organizations, public and private, communities and individuals"

C F Bio-statistics because Bio-statistics is the application of statistics to a wide range of topics in biology.

D T Epidemiology.

E F Statistic because Statistics is the study of the collection, organization, analysis, interpretation, and presentation of data.

20. The purpose of a double blind study

A F Avoid subject bias because Avoid subject bias is only used in a single blind study

B T Avoid observer bias and sampling variation

C F Avoid observer bias because Avoid observer bias is only used in a single blind study

D T Avoid subject bias and doesn't matter for observer because Avoid subject bias and observer.

E T Guard against both experimenter bias and placebo effects.

21. The following vitamin is lost during rice polishing

A F Carotene because the milling and polishing processes both remove important nutrients. A diet based on unenriched white rice leaves people vulnerable to the neurological disease beriberi, due to a deficiency of thiamine (vitamin B_1). White rice is often enriched with some of the nutrients stripped from it during its processing. Enrichment of white rice with B_1, B_3, and iron is required by law in the United States, although these nutrients are only a small portion of what has been removed.

B T Thiamine

C F Cyanocobalamin because the milling and polishing processes both remove important nutrients. A diet based on unenriched white rice leaves people vulnerable to the neurological disease beriberi, due to a deficiency of thiamine (vitamin B_1). White rice is often enriched with some of the nutrients stripped from it during its processing. Enrichment of white rice with B_1, B_3, and iron is required by law in the United States, although these nutrients are only a small portion of what has been removed.

D F Ascorbic Acid because the milling and polishing processes both remove important nutrients. A diet based on unenriched white rice leaves people vulnerable to the neurological disease beriberi, due to a deficiency of thiamine (vitamin B_1). White rice is often enriched with some of the nutrients stripped from it during its processing. Enrichment of white rice with B_1, B_3, and iron is required by law in the United States, although these nutrients are only a small portion of what has been removed.

E F Vitamin E because the milling and polishing processes both remove important nutrients. A diet based on unenriched white rice leaves people vulnerable to the neurological disease beriberi, due to a deficiency of thiamine (vitamin B_1). White rice is often enriched with some of the nutrients stripped from it during its processing. Enrichment of white rice with B_1, B_3, and iron is required by law in the United States, although these nutrients are only a small portion of what has been removed.

22. Double blind study

A F Participant is only not aware of the group allocation and treatment received because participant and investigator are not aware of the group allocation and treatment received.

B T Neither the participant nor the researcher is aware of the group allocation and treatment received.

C F Participant and investigator are aware of the group allocation and treatment received because participant and investigator are not aware of the group allocation and treatment received.

D F Researcher is only not aware of the group allocation and treatment received because participant and investigator are not aware of the group allocation and treatment received.

E F Participant is only aware of the group allocation and treatment received because participant and investigator are not aware of the group allocation and treatment received.

23. Regarding cross-sectional study:

A T Follow up is not a necessary feature.

B F Cause and effect relationship can be established because

C T All cases are seen at one point in time.

D T More useful for chronic diseases.

E T Describes what exists at time of study

24. Regarding the ideal target population in Measles control in emergency situation

A F Routine vaccination because Routine vaccination is not necessary in the emergency situation

B F 14 years and above because 14 years and above is not the ideal target population in the emergency situation

C T 5 years of age.

D T 14 years and below

E T 10 years and above

25. Health education may often fail due to communication barriers between the educator and community. Which of the following is the main communication barrier?

A T Physiological.

B T Psychological.

C T Environmental.

D F Physiological but not Psychological because Physiological and psychological

E F Psychological but not Environmental because Psychological and Environmental

26. To call a person a drug addict, which of the following criteria must be satisfied?

T A Psychological dependence.

T B Physical dependence.

T C Development of tolerance

T D Psychological or physical dependence

T E Dependent on an addictive substance

27. Fat content is highest in:

A F Chicken drumstick because Chicken drumstick contains 4.0g fat

B F Chicken breast because Chicken breast contains 7.0g fat

C T Beef because Beef contains 21.6 g fat

D F Salmon because Salmon contains 11g fat

E T Tuna because Tuna contains 5.1g fat

28. Macronutrient includes

A T Proteins

B T Fats

C T Carbohydrates

D F Iron because is a micro-nutrition's

E F Zinc because is a micro nutrition's

29. Vitamins are a class of

A T Inorganic compounds.

B F Organic compounds because vitamins are classified as inorganic compounds only

C F Either Organic or inorganic compounds because vitamins are classified as inorganic compounds only

D F Neither organic nor inorganic compounds because vitamins are classified as inorganic compounds only

E F Organic and inorganic compounds because vitamins are classified as inorganic compounds only

30. 'A clinically manifest disease of man resulting from an infection' is called:

A T Infectious disease.

B T Contagious disease.

C F Iatrogenic disease because Iatrogenic disease is an inadvertent adverse effect or complication resulting from medical treatment or advice, including that of psychologists, therapists, pharmacists, nurses, physicians, and dentists. Iatrogenesis is not restricted to conventional medicine; it can also result from complementary and alternative medicine treatments.

D F Nosocomial disease because nosocomial disease is an infection whose development is favoured by a hospital environment, such as one acquired by a patient during a hospital visit or one developing among hospital staff. Such infections include fungal and bacterial infections and are aggravated by the reduced resistance of individual patients.

E T Communicable disease

31. 'Number of deaths due to a particular cause (or in a specific age group) per 100 (or 1000) total deaths' is known as:

A F Prevalence rate because the prevalence is calculated by dividing the number of persons with the disease or condition at a particular time point by the number of individuals examined.

B T Proportional mortality rate

C F Case fatality rate because case fatality rate, case fatality ratio or just fatality rate — is the proportion of deaths within a designated population of "cases" (people with a medical condition), over the course of the disease. A CFR is conventionally expressed as a percentage and represents a measure of risk. CFRs are most often used for diseases with discrete, limited time courses, such as outbreaks of acute infections. For example: Assume 9 deaths among 100 people in a community all diagnosed with the same disease. This means that among the 100 people formally diagnosed with the disease, 9 died and 91 recovered. The CFR, therefore, would be 9%. If some of the cases have not yet resolved (either died or recovered) at the time of analysis, this could lead to bias in estimating the CFR.

D F Standardized mortality rate because standardized mortality rate tells how many persons, per thousand of the population, will die in a given year and what the causes of death will be.

E F Incidence rate because Incidence of disease represents the rate of occurrence of new cases arising in a given period in a specified population.

32. A study was conducted in Malaysia with a group of 200 breast cancer patients to determine the quality of life in a single institute. The design of this study is:

A F Case control study because case-control study design should include case and control and match both case and control with certain criteria according to the objectives of the study.

B F Retrospective cohort study because a retrospective cohort study, also called a historic cohort study, (from Latin retr, "look back") generally means to take a look back at events that already have taken place. For example, the term is used in medicine, describing a look back at a patient's medical history or lifestyle. Retrospective cohort studies have existed for approximately as long as prospective cohort studies

C F Concurrent cohort study because Concurrent cohort study is prospective cohort study. A prospective cohort study is a cohort study that follows over time a group of similar individuals (cohorts) who differ with respect to certain factors under study, to determine how these factors affect rates of a certain outcome. For example, one might follow a cohort of middle-aged truck drivers who vary in terms of smoking habits, to test the hypothesis that the 20-year incidence rate of lung cancer will be highest among heavy smokers, followed by moderate smokers, and then nonsmokers.

D T Cross sectional study

E F Descriptive study because Descriptive research, also known as statistical research, describes data and characteristics about the population or phenomenon being studied. However, it does not answer questions about e.g.: how/when/why the characteristics occurred, which is done under analytic research. Although the data description is factual, accurate and systematic, the research cannot describe what caused a situation. Thus, Descriptive research cannot be used to create a *causal relationship*, where one variable affects another. In other words, descriptive research can be said to have a low requirement for internal validity.

33. Highest vitamin A content is seen in:

A F Lemon because 18 IU

B F Apple because 98 IU

C F Tomato because Tomato 1025 IU

D T Spinach because Spinach 2813

E F Broccoli because Broccoli 1207 IU

34. Study of time, place and person distribution of health related events is known as:

A T Descriptive epidemiology

B F Experimental epidemiology because Experimental epidemiology uses an experimental model to confirm a causal relationship suggested by observational studies.

C F Analytical epidemiology because study designed is to investigate hypothesized causal relationships.

D F Clinical epidemiology because Clinical Epidemiology extends the principles of epidemiology to the critical evaluation of diagnostic and therapeutic modalities in clinical practice.

E T Epidemiology

35. If the drug prevent mortality but does not affect cure, then which of the following will be true:

A F Incidence will decrease because prevalence will increase

B F Incidence will increase because prevalence will increase

C F Prevalence will decrease because prevalence will increase

D T Prevalence will increase

E F Incidence and prevalence will increase because prevalence will increase

36. What most describes an abstract of scientific research article

A T The most read section

B F A one- two pages summary of the research because The abstract of a scientific research article should not be more than 300 words

C T Should contain information on minor content of the study.

D F Not contain the key words of the research because The abstract of a scientific research article should contain the keywords of the research

E T Should include the objective of the study

37. Prevalence of a disease

A F Can only be determined by a cohort study because the prevalence is calculated by dividing the number of persons with the disease or condition at a particular time point by the number of individuals examined.

B F Is the number of new cases in a defined population because the prevalence is calculated by dividing the number of persons with the disease or condition at a particular time point by the number of individuals examined.

C T Describes the balance between incidence, mortality and recovery

D F Is the best measure of disease frequency in etiological studies because the prevalence is calculated by dividing the number of persons with the disease or condition at a particular time point by the number of individuals examined.

E T Can determine by cross-sectional study.

38. Vigorous physical activity is bicycling

A F 9 miles per hour because Bicycling 9 miles per hour is considered a moderate physical activity

B T more than 10 miles per hour.

C F less than 10 miles per hour because Bicycling less than 10 miles per hour is also considered a moderate physical activity

D T less than 15 Kilometer per hour.

E T more than 15 Kilometer per hour.

39. The proximate principles food

A T Proteins.

B T Fats.

C T Carbohydrates.

D T Vitamins.

E T Minerals.

40. Assessment methods of nutritional status include

A T Clinical methods

B T Anthropometric methods

C T Biochemical methods.

D T Laboratory Methods

E T Dietary evaluation methods

41. The following is a body building food

A T Grilled chicken

B T Boiled egg

C T Peanut butter

D T Brown rice

E T Cheese

42. The daily fat requirement should be ________ of total daily energy intake?

A F 10% because are less than recommended fat intakes

B F 15% because are less than recommended fat intakes

C T 20%

D F 30% because are more than recommended

E F 40% because are more than recommended

43. The following is/are unsaturated fat

A T Wheat

B T Sunflower

C T Olive

D T Corn

E F Butter because butter is saturated fat

44. The following is essential amino acids

A T Lysine

B F Alanine because alanine is a non-essential amino acid which is synthesized from a pyruvic acid

C T Tryptophan

D T Phenylalanine

E T Leucine

45. Diana is 22 years old, eats and then vomits secretly, What eating disorder does she suffer from?

A F Compulsive overeating because compulsive overeating, also sometimes called food addiction, is characterized by an obsessive relationship to food. Professionals address this with either a behavior therapy model or a food-addiction model

B F Anorexia nervosa because Anorexia nervosa is a persistent, chronic eating disorder characterized by deliberate food restriction and serve, life-threatening weight loss. Anorexia nervosa involves self-starvation motivated by an intense fear of gaining weight along with an extremely distorted body image.

C T Bulimia nervosa

D F Binge eating disorder because Individuals with binge eating disorder gorge like their bulimic counterparts but do not take excessive measures to loss the weight that they gain. Often they are clinically obese. Binge eating episodes are often characterized by eating rapidly, eating large amount of food even when not feeling hungry, and feeling guilty or depressed after overeating.

E F Body dysmorphic disorder because People with body dysmorphic disorder are obsessively concerned with their appearance, and have a distorted view of their own body shape, body size, weight and perceived lack of muscles.

46. 'Keeping the frequency of illness within acceptable limits' is best described as

A F Elimination because Elimination, clearance of a drug or other foreign agent from the body

B F Eradication because Eradication is the reduction of an infectious disease's prevalent in the global host population to zero.

C T Control

D F Surveillance because Surveillance is the monitoring of the behavior, activities, or other changing information, usually of people for the purpose of influencing, managing, directing, or protecting.

E F Observation because Observation is an activity of a living being, such as a human, which is necessary in order to receive knowledge of the world or about the environment through the senses, which often later involves the recording of data via the use of scientific instruments. The term may also refer to any data collected during this activity.

47. What technique of weight assessment is based on the relationship of weight to height?

A F Body consumption index because In physical fitness, body composition is used to describe the percentages of fat, bone and muscle in human bodies.

B T Body mass index

C F Hydrostatic weight because Hydrostatic weighing, also referred to as "underwater weighing," "hydrostatic body composition analysis," and "hydrodensitometry," is a technique for measuring the mass per unit volume of a patient's body.

D F Waist to hip ratio because Waist–hip ratio or waist-to-hip ratio (WHR) is the ratio of the circumference of the waist to that of the hips.

E F Skinfold caliper test because Skinfold caliper is a device which measures the thickness of a fold of your skin with its underlying layer of fat. By doing this at the key locations can be a quite accurate representative of the total amount of fat that is on your body, it is also possible to estimate the total percent of bodyfat on your body.

48. The presence of an infectious agent on a body surface and/or surgical instruments and dressings known as

A F Infection because Infection is the invasion of a host organism's bodily tissues by disease-causing organisms, their multiplication, and the reaction of host tissues to these organisms and the toxins they produce. Infections are caused by microorganisms such as viruses, prions, bacteria, and viroids, and larger organisms like macroparasites and fungi.

B F Infestation because Infestation refers to the state of being invaded or overrun by pests or parasites. It can also refer to the actual organisms living on or within a host.

C T Contamination

D F Pollution because Pollution is the introduction of contaminants into the natural environment that cause adverse change. Pollution can take the form of chemical substances or energy, such as noise, heat or light. Pollutants, the components of pollution, can be either foreign substances/energies or naturally occurring contaminants.

E T Contagion

49. Regarding information in the international death certificate

A T The certificate deals with the immediate and also the underlying cause

B F The certificate deals with the immediate cause only because The standard death certificate should include the bio-data, place of death then cause of death and also the underlying causes.

C F The certificate deals with the underlying cause only because The standard death certificate should include the bio-data, place of death then cause of death and also the underlying causes.

D F Other morbid conditions not related to the cause of death are not included because The standard death certificate should include the bio-data, place of death then cause of death and also the underlying causes.

E T The certificate should include the bio-data

50. The food that is not accepted as a reference protein:

A T Human milk

B T Cow's milk

C F Hen's egg because Hen's egg contains a great variety of nutrients to sustain both life and growth. Egg provides an excellent, inexpensive and low calorie source of high-quality proteins. Moreover, Eggs are a good source of several important nutrients including protein, total fat, monounsaturated fatty acids, polyunsaturated fatty acids, cholesterol, choline, folate, iron, calcium, phosphorus, selenium, zinc and vitamins A, B_2, B_6, B_{12}, D, E and K.

D T Soybean

E T Goat milk

2 PATHOLOGY

2.1 Questions without Answers

1. Regarding granulomatous inflammation
    A. Tuberculosis is a common example
    B. It is characterised by epithelioid cells
    C. It arises secondary to presence of foreign body
    D. Caseation necrosis is commonly seen
    E. There is a predominance of neutrophils.

2. Cells involved in chronic inflammation
    A. macrophages
    B. lymphocytes.
    C. Red blood cells
    D. Epithelioid cells
    E. Endothelial cells

3. Benign tumours are characterised by
    A. Slow growth
    B. Absent of capsule
    C. Metastasis

D. Different histological pattern from parent tissue

E. Absent of marked necrosis within the tumour

4. Common complications of wound healing include

A. Ischemic effect

B. formation of excessive granulation tissue

C. Formation of cancer

D. hypertrophic scar

E. pathological fractures

5. Regarding cancer prognosis

A. Presence of systemic symptoms has bad prognosis

B. Site of the tumour does not affect prognosis

C. Well differentiated tumours have good prognosis

D. Stage 4 tumours are associated with good prognosis

E. Responsiveness to therapy has good prognosis

6. Regarding thrombus

A. The lines of Zahn form a microscopic feature.

B. Red thrombus is characteristic of arterial thrombosis

C. Pulmonary embolism is a complication of venous thrombus

D. It is loosely adherent to vascular endothelium.

E. Reslution is one of the sequelae

7. Morphologic patterns of inflammation

A. Granulomatous inflammation occurs in syphilis.
B. Fibrinous inflammation is commonly seen in serous cavities.
C. Purulent inflammation is charactresticly occurs due to infection by pyogenic bacteria such as staphylococci infection.
D. Serous inflammation characterised by the copious effusion of non-viscous serous fluid, commonly produced by mesothelial cells of serous membranes.
E. Ulcerative inflammation occurrs near an epithelium can result in

the necrotic loss of tissue from the surface.

8. Regarding Hyperpigmentation
   A. Inflammation is a cause
   B. Many forms of hyperpigmentation are caused by an excess production of melanin.
   C. May occurs due to adrenal insufficiency
   D. May occurs after exposure to certain chemicals such as salicylic acid.
   E. Hyperpigmentation can sometimes be induced by dermatological laser procedures.

9. Regarding necrosis
   A. Gangrenous necrosis is seen in the heart
   B. Liquefactive necrosis is common in the brain
   C. Ischemia is the common cause
   D. Protein denaturation is seen in coagulative necrosis
   E. Apoptosis is a type of necrosis

10. Regarding ischemia
    A. It occurs when the blood supply to a tissue is inadequate to meet the tissue's metabolic demands.
    B. Vasculitis is a complication.
    C. Arterial emboli to the brain cause ischemic necrosis of brain tissue.
    D. Ischemic necrosis of the extremities is a serious problem in the hypertension patients.
    E. Atherosclerosis of the major coronary arteries is responsible for the vast majority of the cases of ischemic heart disease.

11. Complications of liver failure include:
    A. Bleeding tendencies
    B. encephalopathy
    C. Esophageal varices
    D. malnutrition
    E. Biliary carcinoma

12. Regarding hepatocellular carcinoma
    A. Hepatitis B virus is implicated in the pathogenesis
    B. The prognosis is good
    C. The liver is cirrhotic in many of the patients
    D. Fibrolamellar type tends to occur in the older age group
    E. Invasion of vascular channels is a feature

13. Regarding chronic pancreatitis
    A. Steatorrhea is a presentation
    B. It can present as episodes of acute inflammation in a previously injured pancreas.
    C. Serum amylase is always elevated
    D. In developed countries, the most common cause is alcohol
    E. Diabetes is a common complication

14. Regarding hepatitis:
    A. Ground glass hepatocytes are characteristic of hepatitis B.
    B. Mallory hyaline is seen in alcoholic hepatitis.
    C. Fibrosis is a hall mark of reversible tissue damage in hepatitis A.
    D. Councilman body is commonly seen in acute hepatitis.
    E. Bridging fibrosis is uncommon in chronic active hepatitis.

15. Regarding Signs and symptoms of Hepatitis B infection:

A. loss of appetite
B. High fever
C. Dark urine
D. nausea
E. vomiting

16. Major risk factors for the development of lung cancer are:

A. helminths
B. cigarette smoking
C. inhalation of asbestos and other dusts
D. pulmonary fibrosis
E. radioactive gases

17. Regarding lung malignancy:

A. Adenocarcinoma is more common in men compared to women
B. Peripheral adenocarcinoma is seen more in non-smokers
C. Small cell carcinoma carries a good prognosis
D. Cough is the most common presentation
E. Squamous cell carcinomas is mostly peripheral in location

18. Regarding bronchiectasis:

A. It complicates acute pneumonia.
B. Bronchial obstruction is commonly predispose to bronchiectasis.
C. Distal bronchi and bronchioles are the most severe involvemened.
D. lung abscess is formed from destruction of bronchial walls.
E. Koilonychia is a presentation

19. Regarding bronchiectasis:
    A. It is reversible abnormal dilatation of bronchi and bronchioles
    B. It is associated with chronic necrotizing infections.
    C. Foreign bodies can predispose to the disease
    D. Purulent sputum is a common symptom
    E. In severe cases significant obstructive ventilatory defects develop.

20. The following are true on chronic bronchitis:
    A. There is infiltration of CD8+ T cells.
    B. The mucosal lining of the larger airways is usually hyperemic.
    C. Microbial infection is often present but plays no role in pathogenesis.
    D. The smoking and irritants induce hypersecretion of the bronchial mucous glands.
    A. The diagnosis of chronic bronchitis is made on clinical grounds.

21. Regarding diabetes mellitus
    A. Type 2 diabetes is more common in children.
    B. Diagnosis is by measurement of HBA_{1c} level.
    C. Hyperthyroidism is a cause.
    D. deposition of amyloid in the islet of Langerhans is seen in type 2 diabetes.
    E. obesity is a predisposing factor for type 2 diabetes.

22. Regarding diabetes mellitus (DM)
    A. Type 2 diabetes mellitus is characterized by loss of the insulin-producing beta cells of the islets of Langerhans in the pancreas
    B. Type 1 diabetes is of the immune-mediated nature
    C. Type 1 diabetes mellitus is characterized by insulin resistance
    D. Gestational diabetes mellitus resembles type 2 diabetes in several respects
    E. Prediabetes indicates a condition that occurs when a person's

blood glucose levels are higher than normal but not high enough for a diagnosis of type 2 DM

23. Regarding acute complications of diabetes mellitus

A. Elevated levels of ketone bodies in the blood decrease the blood's pH leading to diabetic ketoacidosis

B. Severe abdominal pain is common in diabetic ketoacidosis.

C. Hyperosmolar nonketotic state is sharing many symptoms with diabetic ketoacidosis

D. Electrolyte imbalances are common in hyperosmolar nonketotic

E. The patient may become agitated, sweaty, weak in hypoglycemia

24. Causes of Conn syndrome include

A. adrenal carcinoma

B. adrenal hypoplasia

C. Adrenal adenoma

D. dexamethasone-suppressible hyperaldosteronism

E. disorders of the renin-angiotensin system

25. Regarding adrenal diseases:

A. Auto-immune disease is a cause of adrenal hypofunction.

B. Hyperpigmentation occurs in primary adrenal failure.

C. Adrenal insufficiency causes hyponatremia.

D. Hypertension is a feature of Conn's syndrome.

E. Pheochromocytoma causes hypotension.

26. Regarding lipoma

A. It is a malignant tumor composed of adipose tissue

B. Lipomas are commonly found in children

C. Adenolipomas are lipomas associated with eccrine sweat glands

D. Lipomas are usually relatively small with diameters of about 1–3 cm

E. familial multiple lipomatosis is a leading cause

27. Regarding osteosarcoma
    A. It is common in adolescents
    B. If occur in elderly, it is associated with worse prognosis
    C. Chondrosarcoma typically affects children
    D. Ewing sarcoma consists of small cells on histology
    E. Giant cell tumour is seen characteristically around the knee

28. Regarding rheumatoid arthritis
    A. It is an autoimmune disease that affects many tissues and organs
    B. It is monoarthritis disease
    C. There is a genetic link with HLA-DR4 and the disease
    D. X-rays of the hands and feet are generally performed to the patients
    E. A negative rheumatoid factor is enough to exclude the disease

29. Regarding gout
    A. Is a cause of kidney stones
    B. Heart diseases are a risk factor.
    C Is associated with low uric acid level in blood
    D. Sea food is a risk factor
    E. The formation of tophi in the central nervous system is a complication.

30. Regarding systemic lupus erythematosis
    A. It is due to Type III hypersensitivity reaction.
    B. The disease occurs nine times more often in men than in women
    C. Classical skin butterfly rash is characteristic.
    D. Usually causes severe destruction of the joints
    E. Antinuclear antibody test is diagnostic

31. Signs and Symptoms of bladder carcinoma include
    A. Unexplained hematuria (gross or microscopic).
    B. Urinary obstruction
    C. Anemia
    D. Dysuria, burning and frequency
    E. Pelvic pain

32. Signs and Symptoms of Renal cell carcinoma
    A. Gross or microscopic hematuria
    B. A palpable mass
    C. Hypertension
    D. Hypocalcemia
    E. Paraneoplastic syndromes

33. Regarding nephrotic syndrome:
    A. It refers to a clinical complex that includes massive protienuria.
    B Among children it may often be associated with a systemic disease.
    C. The most frequent systemic cause of the nephrotic syndrome is hypertension
    D. The most important of the primary glomerular lesions that lead to nephrotic syndrome are membranous GN, and lipoid nephrosis.
    E. Generalized edema, is the most obvious clinical manifestation.

34. Regarding glomerular diseases
    A. It is one of the most common causes of chronic renal failure
    B. It is induced by antigen-antibody reactions.
    C. Antigen-antibody deposition in the glomerulus is a major pathway of glomerular injury.

D. The loss of glomerular barrier function, is manifested by proteinuria.

E. Epithelial cell injury of glomeruli can be induced by antibodies to visceral epithelial cell antigens.

35. Signs and symptoms of renal stones

A. Excruciating, intermittent pain that radiates from the flank to the groin or to the genital area and inner thigh

B. Urinary urgency

C. Hematuria

D. Hypertension

E. Nausea and vomiting

36. Prognostic factors of breast carcinoma include

A. Tumour size and axillary node status

B. Tumour grade

C. Histologic Subtypes

D. Androgen receptors

E. Molecular Markers

37. Regarding signs and symptoms of breast cancer

A. The first noticeable symptom of breast cancer is typically a lump.

B. Thickening different from the other breast tissue,

C. One breast becoming larger or lower

D. Inverted nipple

E. skin puckering or dimpling

38. Regarding morphology of fibroadenoma

A. Majority of them are less than three centimetres in diameter

B. The tumor is round or ovoid, elastic, and nodular, and has a smooth surface

C. Microscopically: it is a benign tumor composed of two elements : epithelium and stroma.

D. The epithelial proliferation appears in a single terminal ductal unit and describes duct-like spaces surrounded by a fibroblastic stroma

E. In intracanalicular fibroadenoma, there is stromal proliferation predominates and compresses the ducts.

39. Risk factors of prostatic cancer include

A. Older age above 65 year

B. Family history/genetics of prostatic cancer

C. Lack of exercise and a sedentary lifestyle

D. Low calcium intake

E. African-American race

40. Risk factors of ovarian cancer include

A. Personal history of cancer

B. Age over 55

C. Menopausal hormone therapy

D. Older women who have never been pregnant

E. being underweight

41. Regarding Aschoff bodies

A. They are nodules found in the hearts of individuals with chronic heart disease.

B. Fully developed Aschoff bodies are granulomatous structures consisting of fibrinoid change

C. They contain lymphocytic infiltration

D. There are abnormal macrophages surrounding necrotic centres

E. The Aschoff nodules are spheroidal or fusiform distinct tiny structures,

42. Regarding presentations of right sided heart failure

A. Hepatomegaly

B. Splenomegaly

C. Peripheral edema

D. Pleural effusion

E. Low blood pressure

43. Regarding rheumatic fiver

A. It is acute immunologically mediated

B. It is multisystem inflammatory disease

C. It follows an episode of group A srteptococcal pharingitis

D. It often follows streptococcal infection of skin

E. It causes chronic deformity of the large joints

44. Regarding aneurysm

A. Marfan syndrome is one of the causes.

B. Saccular aneurysms : involving a long segment, vary in diameter(up to 20 cm) and in length.

C. Thoracic aortic aneurysms are far more common than abdominal aortic aneurysms

D. The larger the aneurysm, the more likely it is to rupture.

C. Aortic dissection occurs when the innermost lining of the artery tears and blood leaks into the wall of the artery.

45. Regarding hypertension:

A. It is sustained increase in blood pressure

B. Most of cases are secondary type.

C. Polycystic kidney disease is etiological factor

D. It may complicates diabetes.

E. Retinopathy is a clinical presentation

46. Regarding Berry aneurysm
    A. It is the most common type of aneurysm intracranial aneurysm
    B. It is more common in men
    C. Cigarette smoking is a predisposing factor of its development
    D. It is most frequently seen in the posterior portion of the circle of Willis
    E. Rupture of the aneurysm is associated with delayed clinical manifestation

47. Effects of rapidly progressing hydrocephalus include
    A. Increase in head size in adults
    B. Headache
    C. Vomiting
    D. Tachycardia
    E. Papilloedema

48. Cerebrospinal fluid findings in bacterial meningitis include
    A. Increased lymphocytes
    B. Low glucose
    C. Low protein
    D. Decrease pressure
    E. Increase turbidity

49. Complications of cerebral abscesses include:
    A. Meningitis
    B. Intracranial herniation
    C. Focal neurological deficit
    D. Tumor

E. Epilepsy

50. Predisposing factors of central nervous system neoplasms include:

A. Genetic factors.

B. Chemical and viral factors.

C. Radiation.

D. Immunosupression.

E. Obesity.

2.2 Questions with Answers

1. Regarding granulomatous inflammation
T A. Tuberculosis is a common example
T B. It is characterised by epithelioid cells
F C. It arises secondary to presence of foreign body because it could arises from chronic infection like TB.
T D. Caseation necrosis is commonly seen
T E. There is a predominance of neutrophils.

2. Cells involved in chronic inflammation
T A. macrophages
T B. lymphocytes.
F C. Red blood cells because no role for RBC in chronic inflammation.
T D. Epithelioid cells
F E. Endothelial cells because no role of this type of cell in chronic inflammation.

3. Benign tumours are characterised by
T A. Slow growth
F B. Absent of capsule because the capsule is characteristic of benign tumours.
F C. Metastasis because metastasis occurs only in malignant tumours.
F D. Different histological pattern from parent tissue because the cells here are similar to parent tissue cells
T E. Absent of marked necrosis within the tumour

4. Common complications of wound healing include
F A. Ischemic effect because ischemia is not a part of healing process.
T B. formation of excessive granulation tissue

F C. Formation of cancer because cancer will not complicate the healing process

T D. hypertrophic scar

F E. pathological fractures because healing process is not a cause of pathological fracture.

5. Regarding cancer prognosis

T A. Presence of systemic symptoms has bad prognosis

F B. Site of the tumour does not affect prognosis because the site ıffects the tumour prognosis

T C. Well differentiated tumours have good prognosis

F D. Stage 4 tumours are associated with good prognosis because stahge 4 is the last stage of tumour including metastasis.

T E. Responsiveness to therapy has good prognosis

6. Regarding thrombus

F A. The lines of Zahn form a microscopic feature because they are a macroscopical feature.

F B. Red thrombus is characteristic of arterial thrombosis because red thrombus is characteristic of venous thrombosis.

T C. Pulmonary embolism is a complication of venous thrombus

F D. It is loosely adherent to vascular endothelium.

T E. Reslution is one of the sequelae

7. Morphologic patterns of inflammation

T A. Granulomatous inflammation occurs in syphilis.

T B. Fibrinous inflammation is commonly seen in serous cavities.

T C. Purulent inflammation is charactresticly occurs due to infection by pyogenic bacteria such as staphylococci infection.

T D. Serous inflammation characterised by the copious effusion of non-viscous serous fluid, commonly produced by mesothelial cells of serous membranes.

T E. Ulcerative inflammation occurrs near an epithelium can result in the necrotic loss of tissue from the surface.

8. Regarding Hyperpigmentation

T A. Inflammation is a cause

T B. Many forms of hyperpigmentation are caused by an excess production of melanin.

T C. May occurs due to adrenal insufficiency

T D. May occurs after exposure to certain chemicals such as salicylic acid.

T E. Hyperpigmentation can sometimes be induced by dermatological laser procedures.

9. Regarding necrosis

F A. Gangrenous necrosis is seen in the heart because in heart coagulative necrosis

T B. Liquefactive necrosis is common in the brain

T C. Ischemia is the common cause

T D. Protein denaturation is seen in coagulative necrosis

F E. Apoptosis is a type of necrosis because apoptosis is a programmed cell death.

10. Regarding ischemia

T A. It occurs when the blood supply to a tissue is inadequate to meet the tissue's metabolic demands.

F B. Vasculitis is a complication because vascultis is a cause but not complication of ischemia

T C. Arterial emboli to the brain cause ischemic necrosis of brain tissue.

F D. Ischemic necrosis of the extremities is a serious problem in the hypertension patients because it is a serious problem in diabetic patients

T E. Atherosclerosis of the major coronary arteries is responsible for the vast majority of the cases of ischemic heart disease.

11. Complications of liver failure include:

T A. Bleeding tendencies

T B. encephalopathy

T C. Esophageal varices

T D. malnutrition

F E. Biliary carcinoma because liver failure is not a cause of biliary cancer

12. Regarding hepatocellular carcinoma

T A. Hepatitis B virus is implicated in the pathogenesis

F B. The prognosis is good because the prognosis is bad

T C. The liver is cirrhotic in many of the patients

F D. Fibrolamellar type tends to occur in the older age group because it tends tp occur in the young age group.

T E. Invasion of vascular channels is a feature

13. Regarding chronic pancreatitis

T A. Steatorrhea is a presentation

T B. It can present as episodes of acute inflammation in a previously injured pancreas.

F C. Serum amylase is always elevated because it may elevate and may be normal

T D. In developed countries, the most common cause is alcohol

T E. Diabetes is a common complication

14. Regarding hepatitis:

T A. Ground glass hepatocytes are characteristic of hepatitis B.

T B. Mallory hyaline is seen in alcoholic hepatitis.

F C. Fibrosis is a hall mark of reversible tissue damage in hepatitis A because this is ahall mark of hepatitis B

T D. Councilman body is commonly seen in acute hepatitis.

F E. Bridging fibrosis is uncommon in chronic active hepatitis because this is common in this type of hepatitis.

15. Regarding Signs and symptoms of Hepatitis B infection:

T A. loss of appetite

F B. High fever because it is low grade fever.

T C. Dark urine

T D. nausea

T E. vomiting

16. Major risk factors for the development of lung cancer are:

F A. helminthes because helminthes are not a risk factor for lung cancer.

T B. cigarette smoking

T C. inhalation of asbestos and other dusts

T D. pulmonary fibrosis

T E. radioactive gases

17. Regarding lung malignancy:

F A. Adenocarcinoma is more common in men compared to women because it is more common among women than men

T B. Peripheral adenocarcinoma is seen more in non-smokers

F C. Small cell carcinoma carries a good prognosis because this type of cancer is highly aggressive with bad prognosis.

T D. Cough is the most common presentation

F E. Squamous cell carcinomas is mostly peripheral in location because it is mostly central in location.

18. Regarding bronchiectasis:

F A. It complicates acute pneumonia because acute pneumonia wont complicate to bronchiectasis.

T B. Bronchial obstruction is commonly predispose to bronchiectasis.

T C. Distal bronchi and bronchioles are the most severe involvemened.

T D. lung abscess is formed from destruction of bronchial walls.

F E. Koilonychia is a presentation because clubbing of fingers is the presentation.

19. Regarding bronchiectasis:

F A. It is reversible abnormal dilatation of bronchi and bronchioles because it is reversible dilatation of bronchi.

T B. It is associated with chronic necrotizing infections.

T C. Foreign bodies can predispose to the disease

T D. Purulent sputum is a common symptom

T E. In severe cases significant obstructive ventilatory defects develop.

20. The following are true on chronic bronchitis:

T A. There is infiltration of CD8+ T cells.

T B. The mucosal lining of the larger airways is usually hyperemic.

F C. Microbial infection is often present but plays no role in pathogenesis because microbes are not often present.

T D. The smoking and irritants induce hypersecretion of the bronchial mucous glands.

T A. The diagnosis of chronic bronchitis is made on clinical grounds.

21. Regarding diabetes mellitus

F A. Type 2 diabetes is more common in children becayse type 1 is more common among children

F B. Diagnosis is by measurement of HBA_{1c} level because this test is for monitoring DM but not for diagnosis

T C. Hyperthyroidism is a cause.

T D. deposition of amyloid in the islet of Langerhans is seen in type 2 diabetes.

T E. obesity is a predisposing factor for type 2 diabetes.

22. Regarding diabetes mellitus (DM)

F A. Type 2 diabetes mellitus is characterized by loss of the insulin-producing beta cells of the islets of Langerhans in the pancreas because this is the definition of type 1 DM.

T B. Type 1 diabetes is of the immune-mediated nature

F C. Type 1 diabetes mellitus is characterized by insulin resistance because type 2 is characterized by insulin resistance.

T D. Gestational diabetes mellitus resembles type 2 diabetes in several respects

T E. Prediabetes indicates a condition that occurs when a person's blood glucose levels are higher than normal but not high enough for a diagnosis of type 2 DM

23. Regarding acute complications of diabetes mellitus

T A. Elevated levels of ketone bodies in the blood decrease the blood's pH leading to diabetic ketoacidosis

T B. Severe abdominal pain is common in diabetic ketoacidosis.

T C. Hyperosmolar nonketotic state is sharing many symptoms with diabetic ketoacidosis

T D. Electrolyte imbalances are common in hyperosmolar nonketotic

T E. The patient may become agitated, sweaty, weak in hypoglycemia

24. Causes of Conn syndrome include

T A. adrenal carcinoma

F B. adrenal hypoplasia because adrenal hyperplesia is a cause.

T C. Adrenal adenoma

T D. dexamethasone-suppressible hyperaldosteronism

T E. disorders of the renin-angiotensin system

25. Regarding adrenal diseases:

T A. Auto-immune disease is a cause of adrenal hypofunction.

T B. Hyperpigmentation occurs in primary adrenal failure.

T C. Adrenal insufficiency causes hyponatremia.

T D. Hypertension is a feature of Conn's syndrome.

F E. Pheochromocytoma causes hypotension because it causes hypertension.

26. Regarding lipoma

T A. It is a malignant tumor composed of adipose tissue

F B. Lipomas are commonly found in children because they are commonly found in adults.

T C. Adenolipomas are lipomas associated with eccrine sweat glands

T D. Lipomas are usually relatively small with diameters of about 1–3 cm

T E. familial multiple lipomatosis is a leading cause

27. Regarding osteosarcoma

T A. It is common in adolescents

T B. If occur in elderly, it is associated with worse prognosis

F C. Chondrosarcoma typically affects children because they typically affects adults.

T D. Ewing sarcoma consists of small cells on histology

T E. Giant cell tumour is seen characteristically around the knee

28. Regarding rheumatoid arthritis

T A. It is an autoimmune disease that affects many tissues and organs

F B. It is monoarthritis disease because it is a multi-arthritis disease.

T C. There is a genetic link with HLA-DR4 and the disease

T D. X-rays of the hands and feet are generally performed to the patients

F E. A negative rheumatoid factor is enough to exclude the disease because rheumatoid factor is not a diagnostic test and it could be negative.

29. Regarding gout

T A. Is a cause of kidney stones

F B. Heart diseases are a risk factor because heart disease is complication

F C Is associated with low uric acid level in blood because it is associated with high uric acid.

T D. Sea food is a risk factor

F E. The formation of tophi in the central nervous system is a complication.

30. Regarding systemic lupus erythematosis

T A. It is due to Type III hypersensitivity reaction.

F B. The disease occurs nine times more often in men than in women because it occurs more often among women more than men like other autoimmune disease.

T C. Classical skin butterfly rash is characteristic.

F D. Usually causes severe destruction of the joints because this happens only in rheumatoid arthritis but not SLE.

T E. Antinuclear antibody test is diagnostic

31. Signs and Symptoms of bladder carcinoma include

T A. Unexplained hematuria (gross or microscopic).

T B. Urinary obstruction

T C. Anemia

T D. Dysuria, burning and frequency

T E. Pelvic pain

32. Signs and Symptoms of Renal cell carcinoma

T A. Gross or microscopic hematuria

T B. A palpable mass

T C. Hypertension

F D. Hypocalcemia because hypercalcemia is a presentation.

T E. Paraneoplastic syndromes

33. Regarding nephrotic syndrome:

T A. It refers to a clinical complex that includes massive protienuria.

F B Among children it may often be associated with a systemic disease because among adults is often associated with systemic disease.

F C. The most frequent systemic cause of the nephrotic syndrome is hypertension because diabetes mellitus is the most frequent cause.

T D. The most important of the primary glomerular lesions that lead to nephrotic syndrome are membranous GN, and lipoid nephrosis.

T E. Generalized edema, is the most obvious clinical manifestation.

34. Regarding glomerular diseases

T A. It is one of the most common causes of chronic renal failure

T B. It is induced by antigen-antibody reactions.

T C. Antigen-antibody deposition in the glomerulus is a major pathway of glomerular injury.

T D. The loss of glomerular barrier function, is manifested by proteinuria.

T E. Epithelial cell injury of glomeruli can be induced by antibodies to visceral epithelial cell antigens.

35. Signs and symptoms of renal stones

T A. Excruciating, intermittent pain that radiates from the flank to the groin or to the genital area and inner thigh

T B. Urinary urgency

T C. Hematuria

F D. Hypertension because renal stone will not cause hypertension

T E. Nausea and vomiting

36. Prognostic factors of breast carcinoma include

T A. Tumour size and axillary node status

T B. Tumour grade

T C. Histologic Subtypes

F D. Androgen receptors because estrogen receptors are the prognostic factor.

T E. Molecular Markers

37. Regarding signs and symptoms of breast cancer

T A. The first noticeable symptom of breast cancer is typically a lump.

T B. Thickening different from the other breast tissue,

T C. One breast becoming larger or lower

T D. Inverted nipple

T E. skin puckering or dimpling

38. Regarding morphology of fibroadenoma

T A. Majority of them are less than three centimetres in diameter

T B. The tumor is round or ovoid, elastic, and nodular, and has a smooth surface

T C. Microscopically: it is a benign tumor composed of two elements : epithelium and stroma.

T D. The epithelial proliferation appears in a single terminal ductal unit and describes duct-like spaces surrounded by a fibroblastic stroma

T E. In intracanalicular fibroadenoma, there is stromal proliferation predominates and compresses the ducts.

39. Risk factors of prostatic cancer include

T A. Older age above 65 year

T B. Family history/genetics of prostatic cancer

T C. Lack of exercise and a sedentary lifestyle

F D. Low calcium intake because the high calcium intake is the risk factor.

T E. African-American race

40. Risk factors of ovarian cancer include

T A. Personal history of cancer

T B. Age over 55

T C. Menopausal hormone therapy

T D. Older women who have never been pregnant

F E. being underweight because obesity is a risk factor

41. Regarding Aschoff bodies

F A. They are nodules found in the hearts of individuals with chronic heart disease because they are characteristics of acute rheumatic fever.

T B. Fully developed Aschoff bodies are granulomatous structures consisting of fibrinoid change

T C. They contain lymphocytic infiltration

T D. There are abnormal macrophages surrounding necrotic centres

T E. The Aschoff nodules are spheroidal or fusiform distinct tiny structures,

42. Regarding presentations of right sided heart failure

T A. Hepatomegaly

T B. Splenomegaly

T C. Peripheral edema

T D. Pleural effusion

F E. Low blood pressure because high blood pressure is a presentation of RHF.

43. Regarding rheumatic fiver

T A. It is acute immunologically mediated

T B. It is multisystem inflammatory disease

T C. It follows an episode of group A srteptococcal pharingitis

F D. It often follows streptococcal infection of skin because it often follows streptococcal pharyngitis.

F E. It causes chronic deformity of the large joints because the joint lesion is reversible and subside after awhile .

44. Regarding aneurysm

T A. Marfan syndrome is one of the causes.

F. B. Saccular aneurysms : involving a long segment, vary in diameter(up to 20 cm) and in length because this definitions of fusiform type.

F C. Thoracic aortic aneurysms are far more common than abdominal aortic aneurysms because the abdominal aortic aneurysms are the most common type.

T D. The larger the aneurysm, the more likely it is to rupture.

T C. Aortic dissection occurs when the innermost lining of the artery tears and blood leaks into the wall of the artery.

45. Regarding hypertension:

T A. It is sustained increase in blood pressure

F B. Most of cases are secondary type because the most of cases are essential type HT.

T C. Polycystic kidney disease is etiological factor

T D. It may complicates diabetes.

T E. Retinopathy is a clinical presentation

46. Regarding Berry aneurysm

T A. It is the most common type of aneurysm intracranial aneurysm

F B. It is more common in men

T C. Cigarette smoking is a predisposing factor of its development

F D. It is most frequently seen in the posterior portion of the circle of Willis because it is most seen in the anterior portion of circle of willis

F E. Rupture of the aneurysm is associated with delayed clinical manifestation because the rapture associated with sudden clinical manifestations.

47. Effects of rapidly progressing hydrocephalus include

F A. Increase in head size in adults because this occurs in children

T B. Headache

T C. Vomiting

F D. Tachycardia because it is bradycardia

T E. Papilloedema

48. Cerebrospinal fluid findings in bacterial meningitis include

F A. Increased lymphocytes because there is decreased lymphocytes.

T B. Low glucose

F C. Low protein because protein is high

F D. Decrease pressure because there is high pressure.

T E. Increase turbidity

49. Complications of cerebral abscesses include:

T A. Meningitis

T B. Intracranial herniation

T C. Focal neurological deficit

F D. Tumor because abscess wont leads to brain tumours

T E. Epilepsy

50. Predisposing factors of central nervous system neoplasms include:

T A. Genetic factors.

T B. Chemical and viral factors.

T C. Radiation.

T D. Immunosupression.

F E. Obesity because obesity is not recorded as predisposing factor for CNS tumours.

3 PHARMACOLOGY

3.1 Questions without Answers

1. Bioavailability of a drug is nearly 100% when given by following route:

	A	Oral
	B	Intravenous
	C	Subcutaneous
	D	Inhalation
	E	Rectal

2. Drug absorption is satisfactory when:

	A	Molecular size & shape is small.
	B	Water solubility is high.
	C	Drug is ionized poorly
	D	Food is present in the stomach
	E	Lipid solubility is high

3. Protein bound drugs are:

	A	Biologically active
	B	Biologically inactive
	C	Rapidly excreted
	D	Readily penetrate cell membrane
	E	Rapidly metabolism

4. The first pharmacokinetic drug profile is:

	A	Metabolism
	B	Excretion
	C	Distribution
	D	Absorption
	E	Plasma protein binding

5. Regarding the following drugs undergoing hepatic first pass metabolism is:

	A	Nicotine
	B	Stilbesterol
	C	Chlorpromazine
	D	Propranolol
	E	Diazepam

6. Regarding pharmacodynamics of drugs is

	A	To improve Efficacy and safety of drug therapy
	B	To the ideal pharmacological action
	C	To avoid the serous side effect
	D	To avoid or minimise drug interactions
	E	To the ideal dose of drug

7. Regarding an agonist

	A	Any substance that brings about a change in biologic function through its chemical action.
	B	A specific regulatory molecule in the biologic system where a drug interacts.
	C	A drug that binds to a receptor and stimulates cellular activity.
	D	A drug that binds to a receptor and inhibits or opposes cellular activity.
	E	A drug directed at parasites infecting the patient.

8. Which of the following can produce a therapeutic response? A drug that is:

	A	Bound to plasma albumin
	B	Concentrated in the bile
	C	Concentrated in the urine
	D	Not absorbed from the GI tract
	E	Unbound to plasma proteins

9. A competitive antagonist affects the agonist ____ and a non-competitive antagonist affect the agonist ____.

	A	Potency; Efficacy
	B	Efficacy; Potency
	C	Duration; onsite
	D	onsite; Duration
	E	Absorption; elimination

10. Which of the following would occur with an antagonist binding to a receptor and not an agonist?

	A	Ion channel closed
	B	Enzyme inhibited
	C	Endogenous mediator blocked
	D	Ion channel modulated
	E	DNA transcription

11.Which of the following is NOT a second messenger associated with G proteins?

	A	DAG
	B	GDP
	C	IP3
	D	cAMP
	E	cGMP

12. Drugs which have effects on ANS are

	A	Work on sympathetic and parasympathetic nervous system
	B	Work only on sympathetic nervous system
	C	Work only on parasympathetic nervous system
	D	directly work on Adrenoreceptors only
	E	directly work only on Adrenoreceptors and parasympathetic receptors

13. Drugs that stimulate directly Adrenoreceptors only are,

	A	Sympathomimetic drugs
	B	Direct sympathomimetic drugs
	C	Indirect sympathomimetic rugs
	D	Parasympathomimetic drugs
	E	Direct Parasympathomimetic drugs

14. Drugs that block directly Adrenoreceptors only are,

	A	Sympathomimetic drugs
	B	Direct sympathomimetic drugs
	C	Indirect sympathomimetic rugs
	D	Direct sympatholytic drugs
	E	Direct parasympatholytic drugs

15. Drugs that produce responses like catecholamines without interact with their receptors can be called

	A	Sympathomimetic drugs
	B	Direct sympathomimetic drugs
	C	Indirect sympathomimetic drugs
	D	Indirect sympatholytics drugs
	E	Parasympathomimetics

16. The indirect sympathomimetic drugs mode of action include

	A	Inhibition of catecholamine metabolism at synaptic cleft
	B	Inhibition of catecholamine uptake by nerve terminal
	C	Catecholamine secretion
	D	Depletion of catecholamine storage
	E	Stimulate adrenergic receptors

17. Regarding selectivity of β-blocker drug is important issue in clinical uses

	A	In hypertensive patient with diabetes mellitus
	B	In hypertension patient with asthma
	C	In hypertensive patient with heart disease
	D	In hypertensive patient with liver disease
	E	In hypertensive patient with kidney disease

18. True regarding intrinsic activity of β-blocker drug is

	A	The capacity to activate the receptors in the process of the drug-receptor interaction.
	B	Important when used for heart diseases
	C	Important when used for asthma
	D	Important when used for treatment of hypertension
	E	Contraindicated in angina disease

19. Drugs that activate cholinorceptors are,

	A	Parasympathomimetic drugs
	B	Direct parasympathomimetic drugs
	C	Indirect parasympathomimetic drugs
	D	Direct sympathomimetics
	E	Indirect sympathomimetics

20. Drugs that inactivate cholinoreceptors are,

	A	Parasympathomimetic drugs
	B	Direct parasympathomimetic drugs
	C	Indirect parasympathomimetic rugs
	D	Direct parasympatholytic drugs
	E	Antagonist agent

21. Drugs that produce responses like acetylcholine without interact with their receptors are

	A	Paraympathomimetic drugs
	B	Direct parasympathomimetic drugs
	C	Indirect parasympathomimetic drugs
	D	Indirect parasympatholytics drugs
	E	Indirect sympathomimetics

22. The indirect parasympathomimatic drugs mode of action include

	A	Inhibition of acetylcholine metabolism at synaptic cleft
	B	Inhibition of acetylcholine uptake by nerve terminal
	C	Acetylcholine secretion
	D	Depletion of acetylcholine storage
	E	Increase Ach synthesis

23. The clinical use of muscarinic agonists include

	A	in treating glaucoma
	B	in treating asthma
	C	in treating heart failure
	D	in treating constipation
	E	assist bladder emptying

24. The clinical use of muscarinic antagonists include

	A	treating urinary incontinence
	B	in treating asthma
	C	in treating diarrhea
	D	treat of glaucoma
	E	treat of hypertension

25. unwanted effects of muscarinic antagonists, such as

	A	Dry mouth
	B	Constipation
	C	Blurred vision
	D	Near vision is impaired
	E	Increase fluid secretion

26. Urinary retention in elderly men with prostatic enlargement can treated by

	A	muscarinic antagonists
	B	muscarinic agonists
	C	indirect Parasympathomimetic
	D	alpha blocker
	E	antiandorgenic drugs

27. Indirect cholinomimetic drug is;

	A	d-tubocurarine
	B	atropine
	C	pilocarpine
	D	physostigmine
	E	neostigmine

28. Muscarinic receptor activation causes all the following EXCEPT

	A	stimulation of inositol triphosphate signal transducing mechanism
	B	activation of potassium channel
	C	opening of sodium channel
	D	release of nitric oxide from endothelial cells
	E	open Ca^{2+} channel

29. Intraocular administration of 1% acetylcholine produces:

	A	contraction of ciliary muscle.
	B	reduction of intraocular pressure.
	C	stimulation of lacrimal secretion.
	D	transient miosis.
	E	Transient mydriases

30. The preferred cholinergic agonist in post operative urinary retention is:

	A	bethanechol.

	B	arecoline.
	C	acetylcholine
	D	physostigmine
	E	atropine

31. Which of the following is NOT a clinical feature of acute belladona poisoning?

	A	copious salivation
	B	urgency for urination but difficult to urinate
	C	tachycardia
	D	delirium
	E	constipation

32. Abrupt withdrawal of clonidine after chronic use causes:

	A	rise of the blood pressure
	B	increase heart rate
	C	bronchoconstriction
	D	constipation
	E	increase intraocular pressure

33. The substances produced locally by one group of cells and exert effects on other types of cells in the same regionare,

	A	Called Autacoids

	B	Called also local hormones
	C	Work only on parasympathetic nervous system
	D	Some of analogue clinically used for prevention
	E	They act through cell membrane receptors

34. The antagonist drugs which work on autacoids pathway used for treatment of

	A	Migraine and pain
	B	Inflammatory
	C	Asthma
	D	Vomiting
	E	Allergic reaction

35. True regarding to histamine

	A	Is synthesized locally form the amino acid histidine
	B	Orally inactive
	C	Receptors are G-protein coupled receptors
	D	Antihistamine drugs compete on H1 receptor
	E	Histamine analogue used in treat vertigo in Miniere's disease

36. Serotonin (5-hydroxytryptamine),

	A	Is localized in the intestines, platelets

	B	Is Synthesised from the amino acid tryptophan
	C	Is Metabolised by a monoamine oxidise, adehydrogenase, and decarboxliase
	D	Has cell membrane receptors belong to G-protein
	E	In CNS is considered as neurotransmitter

37. True regarding *Eicosanoids*

	A	Are parts of autacoids mediators
	B	Include Prostaglandins and Leukotrienes
	C	Are polyunsaturated essential fatty acids
	D	Are synthesised by phospholipase A, cyclo-oxygenase (COX) and lipooxyganse
	E	The half-life of most prostaglandins in the circulation is less than 1 minute.

38. True regarding prostanoids

	A	Encompasse the prostaglandins and the thromboxanes
	B	Prostanoid receptors which are typical G-protein-coupled receptors
	C	Causes bronchoconstriction
	D	Used in gastric ulcer
	E	In treatment of allergy

39. True regarding therapeutic uses of prostanoid analogues

	A	Termination of pregnancy and induction of labour
	B	To prevent ulcers associated with NSAD
	C	Treatment of glaucoma
	D	To prevent platelet aggregation
	E	Auto immune disease

40. True regarding leukotrienes

	A	Are synthesised from arachidonic acid by lipoxygenase-catalysed pathways.
	B	Receptors utilise inositol trisphosphate and increased cytosolic Ca^{2+}
	C	are potent spasmogens
	D	cause an increase in mucus secretion
	E	fall in blood pressure

41. True regarding leukotrenes Antagonist

	A	used in treatment of asthma
	B	zafirlukast and montelukast are direct leukotrine antagonist.
	C	Zileuton is indirect of leukotreine blocker
	D	Important when used for treatment of hypertension
	E	Zileuton inhibits lipoxygenase enzyme

42. True regarding chemotherapy

	A	Is designed to inhibit/kill the infecting organism and to have no/minimal effect on the recipient.
	B	Is designed to inhibit/kill the infecting organism and to have effect on the recipient.
	C	Treatment of systemic infections with specific drugs that selectively suppress the infecting microorganism without significantly affecting the host.
	D	Treatment of systemic infections with specific drugs that selectively suppress the infecting microorganism without significantly affecting the host.
	E	

43. General principles of antimicrobial use are:

	A	It is not to be prescribed indiscriminately.
	B	Rapidly acting and selective drugs to be used wherever possible
	C	It is prescribed for any types of infectious conditions.
	D	Broad-spectrum are used when a specific one cannot be determined or not suitable.
	E	It is stopped immediately when symptoms of infection disappear.

44.True regarding therapeutic index (TI) of antimicrobials

	A	penicillins, some cephalosporins and erythromycin have high therapeutic index
	B	Aminoglycosides, tetracyclines and chloramphenicol have low therapeutic index
	C	Polymyxin B, vancomycin and amphotericin B have very low therapeutic index
	D	Antibiotic with high TI can be prescribed for pregnant women
	E	Antibiotic with low TI can be prescribed for pregnant women

45.True regarding resistance

	A	It refers to unresponsiveness of a microorganism to an antimicrobial drugs
	B	Natural resistance does not pose a significant clinical problem.
	C	Natural resistance does pose a significant clinical problem.
	D	Acquired resistance poses a significant clinical problem
	E	Cross resistance does not pose a significant clinical problem

46. True regarding Prevention of drug resistance

	A	No indiscriminate and inadequate or unduly prolonged use of AMAs
	B	Rapidly acting and selective (narrowspectrum) AMAs whenever possible

	C	Use combination of AMAs whenever prolonged therapy is undertake
	D	Use broad-spectrum drugs
	E	Antimicrobial is prescribed after sensitivity test

47.True combined use of antimicrobial drugs

	A	To achieve synergism
	B	To achieve potency
	C	To reduce severity of adverse effects
	D	To prevent of resistance
	E	To broden the spectrum of antimicrobial action

48.True regarding failure of antimicrobial therapy

	A	Improper selection of drug, dose, route or duration of treatment.
	B	Treatment begun too late
	C	Failure to take necessary adjuvant measures
	D	Poor host defence
	E	Presence of dormant or altered organisms

49. Use the accompanied diagram for the following questions:

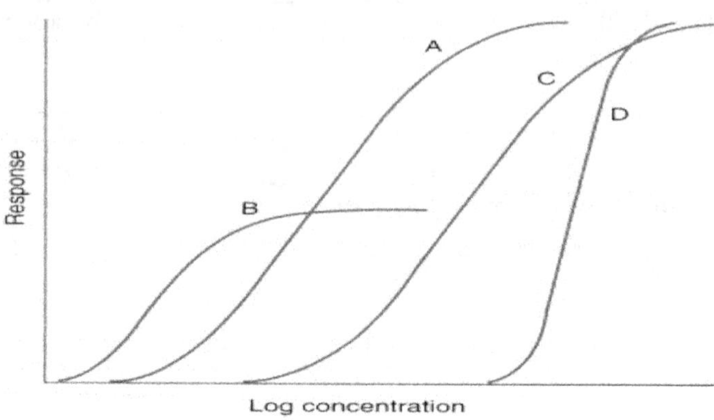

49.1) Which of the following drugs would require the most care when administrating, if the upper portion of the dose-response curve signified severe toxicity?

	A	A
	B	B
	C	C
	D	D

49.2) Which drug is the least efficacious?

	A	A
	B	B
	C	C
	D	D

49.3) Intrinsic activity is a drug's ability to elicit:

	A	Strong receptor binding
	B	Weak receptor binding
	C	Response
	D	Excretion
	E	Distribution

49.4) Which direction would a partial agonist shift the dose-response curve when compared to a full agonist?

	A	To the left
	B	To the right
	C	Down
	D	Up
	E	To the right and possibly down

49.5) Which direction would a competitive antagonist (plus agonist) shift the dose response curve when compared to a full agonist?

	A	To the left
	B	To the right
	C	Down
	D	Up
	E	To the right and possibly down

3.2 Questions with Answers

1. Bioavailability of a drug is nearly 100% when given by following route:

F	A	Oral because oral route not all the dug can be absorbed because due to GIT factors or liver enzymes metabolise drug.
T	B	Intravenous
F	C	Subcutaneous because subcutaneous also not all drug can be absorbed either due to skin factors such blood circulation or enzymes metabolise drug.
F	D	Inhalation because inhalation normally not use for systemic effect it used for local effects. Even though it can be used for systemic effect such general anaesthesia such as NO which has gas property.
F	E	Rectal because rectal drug is required absorption to rich blood circulation.

2. Drug absorption is satisfactory when:

T	A	Molecular size & shape is small.
F	B	Water solubility is high because any molecule to be absorbed through the biological membrane lipid solubility is required because cell membrane is consisting of lipid.
T	C	Drug is ionized poorly
F	D	Food is present in the stomach because food when present in stomach it will dilly stomach empty at the same time it will combite with drug molecules on site of absorption.
T	E	Lipid solubility is high

3. Protein bound drugs are:

F	A	Biologically active because Only the free form of drug molecule will be active biologically.
T	B	Biologically inactive
F	C	Rapidly excreted because Drug to be execrated should be first metabolised and drug cannot metabolism unless in free from.
F	D	Readily penetrate cell membrane because cannot penetrate the cell membrane because it will not has enough lipid solubility.
T	E	Rapidly metabolism

4. The first pharmacokinetic drug profile is:

F	A	Metabolism because metabolism is not the first pharmacokinetics and is occurred after absorption.
F	B	Excretion because excretion is occurred after absorption and metabolism.
F	C	Distribution because distribution occurs after absorption
T	D	Absorption
F	E	Plasma protein binding because plasma protein binding occurs after absorption and during distribution when drug molecules reach to blood circulation.

5. TRUE regarding the following drugs undergoing hepatic first pass metabolism is:

F	A	Nicotine because Nicotine is taken through respiratory system
F	B	Stilbesterol because Stilbesterol has not metabolism before inter blood circulation
F	C	Chlorpromazine because Chlorpromazine has not metabolism before inter blood circulation.

T	D	Propranolol
T	E	Diazepam

6. Regarding pharmacodynamics of drugs is

T	A	To improve Efficacy and safety of drug therapy
T	B	To the ideal pharmacological action
T	C	To avoid the serous side effect
T	D	To avoid or minimise drug interactions
F	E	To the ideal dose of drug because Pharmacodynamics of drug not dependant on ideal dose.

7. Regarding an agonist

F	A	Any substance that brings about a change in biologic function through its chemical action because Chemical reaction is not the mode of action of agonist in biological siting
F	B	A specific regulatory molecule in the biologic system where a drug interacts because Agonist it will stimulate the function of cells in this statement not mention about it.
T	C	A drug that binds to a receptor and stimulates cellular activity.
F	D	A drug that binds to a receptor and inhibits or opposes cellular activity because Agonist it will stimulate the function of cells support the cellular activity
F	E	A drug directed at parasites infecting the patient because The tissue turgget for agonist will be part of body.

8. Which of the following can produce a therapeutic response? A drug that is:

F	A	Bound to plasma albumin because Only for free form
F	B	Concentrated in the bile because Only during elimination if through liver
F	C	Concentrated in the urine because Only during elimination if through kidney
F	D	Not absorbed from the GI tract because Will be no response if drug not reach to site of action
T	E	Unbound to plasma proteins

9. A competitive antagonist affects the agonist ____ and a non-competitive antagonist affect the agonist ____.

T	A	Potency; Efficacy
F	B	Efficacy; Potency Concentration play the main factor when the concentration of agonist increase will maintain the effect in the present of competitive antagonist. In order to maintain the concentration agonist we have to increase the dose. The dose of drug is related to the potency of durg. In non-compititaive antagonist the concentration will not the main factors to maintain the effect of agonist. The main factors will be the antagonist. The end effect of non-copetitive is reduce the efficacy of agonist.
F	C	Duration; onsite There are no relation on duration of action and onsite of action of agonist when antagonist is present.
F	D	onsite; Duration There are no relation on duration of action and onsite of action of agonist when antagonist is present.

F	E	Absorption; elimination There are no relation on absorption and elimination of agonist when antagonist is present.

10. Which of the following would occur with an antagonist binding to a receptor and not an agonist?

F	A	Ion channel closed because Antagonist is a type of receptor ligand or drug that does not provoke a biological response itself upon binding to a receptor. Based on that all the option are not correct except C
F	B	Enzyme inhibited because Antagonist is a type of receptor ligand or drug that does not provoke a biological response itself upon binding to a receptor. Based on that all the option are not correct except C
T	C	Endogenous mediator blocked
F	D	Ion channel modulated because Antagonist is a type of receptor ligand or drug that does not provoke a biological response itself upon binding to a receptor. Based on that all the option are not correct except C
F	E	DNA transcription because Antagonist is a type of receptor ligand or drug that does not provoke a biological response itself upon binding to a receptor. Based on that all the option are not correct except C

11.Which of the following is NOT a second messenger associated with G proteins?

F	A	DAG because DAG and IP3 is 2nd messenger associated with G protein which stimulate phospholipase A2
T	B	GDP
F	C	IP3 because DAG and IP3 is 2nd messenger associated with G protein which stimulate phospholipase A2

F	D	cAMP because cAMP is 2nd messenger associated with G protein which stimulate adenylyl cyclise enzyme
F	E	cGMP because cGMP is2nd messenger associated with G protein which stimulate Guanylate cyclase

12. Drugs which have effects on ANS are

T	A	Work on sympathetic and parasympathetic nervous system
F	B	Work only on sympathetic nervous system because Sympathetic nervous system is part of ANS
F	C	Work only on parasympathetic nervous system because Parasympathetic nervous system is part of ANS
F	D	directly work on Adrenoreceptors only because Drugs work direct or indirect on both Adrenoreceptors and parasympathetic receptors
F	E	directly work only on Adrenoreceptors and parasympathetic receptors because Drugs work direct or indirect

13. Drugs that stimulate directly Adrenoreceptors only are,

T	A	Sympathomimetic drugs
T	B	Direct sympathomimetic drugs
T	C	Indirect sympathomimetic rugs
F	D	Parasympathomimetic drugs because Parasympathomimetic which drugs stimulate paroreceptors (N & M receptors) or faceletate Ach secretion
F	E	Direct Parasympathomimetic drugs because Direct Parasympathomimetic drugs which drugs stimulate

		paroreceptors (N & M receptors)

14. Drugs that block directly Adrenoreceptors only are,

F	A	Sympathomimetic drugs because A sympathomimetic which drug can stimulate adrenoreceptors directly or facilitated catecholamine secretion.
F	B	Direct sympathomimetic drugs because Direct sympathomimetic which drugs stimulate adrenoreceptors directly not block
F	C	Indirect sympathomimetic rugs because indirect sympathomimetic which drugs facilitated catecholamine secretion
T	D	Direct sympatholytic drugs
F	E	Direct parasympatholytic drugs because are drug which block parasympathetic receptors (N & M receptors)

15. Drugs that produce responses like catecholamines without interact with their receptors can be called

T	A	Sympathomimetic drugs
T	B	Direct sympathomimetic drugs
F	C	Indirect sympathomimetic drugs
F	D	Indirect sympatholytics drugs
F	E	Parasympathomimetics

16. The indirect sympathomimetic drugs mode of action include

T	A	Inhibition of catecholamine metabolism at synaptic cleft
T	B	Inhibition of catecholamine uptake by nerve terminal
T	C	Catecholamine secretion
F	D	Depletion of catecholamine storage because Are drugs have opposite effect to catecholamine
F	E	Stimulate adrenergic receptors because direct sympathomimetic

17. Regarding selectivity of β-blocker drug is important issue in clinical uses

T	A	In hypertensive patient with diabetes mellitus
T	B	In hypertension patient with asthma
T	C	In hypertensive patient with heart disease
F	D	In hypertensive patient with liver disease because using β-blocker drug for treatment hypertension will not mask symptom or increase symptom lead to serious out come.but it may affect drug duration of action either decrease or increase based on the liver condition. The most common is increase drug duration of action. This problem can be increase the interval time or the dose.
F	E	In hypertensive patient with kidney disease because using β-blocker drug for treatment hypertension will not mask symptom or increase symptom lead to serious out come.but it may affect drug duration of action either decrease or increase based on the liver condition. The most common is increase drug duration of action. This problem can be increase the interval time or the

		dose.

18. Regarding intrinsic activity of β-blocker drug is

T	A	The capacity to activate the receptors in the process of the drug-receptor interaction.
T	B	Important when used for heart diseases
F	C	Important when used for asthma because β-blocker drug not used for treatment of asthma
F	D	Important when used for treatment of hypertension because intrinsic activity of β-blocker will not add any advantages
T	E	Contraindicated in angina disease

19. Drugs that activate cholinorceptors are,

F	A	Parasympathomimetic drugs because Parasympathomimetic drugs can be drug activate cholinorceptors or facilitate Ach secretion
T	B	Direct parasympathomimetic drugs
F	C	Indirect parasympathomimetic drugs because Indirect parasympathomimetic which drugs facilitate Ach secretion
F	D	Direct sympathomimetics because Direct sympathomimetics drug activate adrenoreceptors
F	E	Indirect sympathomimetics because Indirect sympathomimetics which drugs facilitate AN and NA secretion

20. Drugs that inactivate cholinoreceptors are,

F	A	Parasympathomimetic drugs because Drug activate cholinoreceptors or facilitated Ach secretion or decrease Ach metabolism
F	B	Direct parasympathomimetic drugs because Drug that activate cholinoreceptors
F	C	Indirect parasympathomimetic rugs because Drugs that facilitate Ach secretion or decrease Ach metabolism
T	D	Direct parasympatholytic drugs
T	E	Antagonist agent

21. Drugs that produce responses like acetylcholine without interact with their receptors are

F	A	Paraympathomimetic drugs because Drugs show like Ach with and without interact with their receptors
F	B	Direct parasympathomimetic drugs because Drugs show like Ach with interact with their receptors
T	C	Indirect parasympathomimetic drugs
F	D	Indirect parasympatholytics drugs because Drugs block Ach effect
F	E	Indirect sympathomimetics because Drugs show AN & NA like effect not Ach

22. The indirect parasympathomimatic drugs mode of action include

T	A	Inhibition of acetylcholine metabolism at synaptic cleft
F	B	Inhibition of acetylcholine uptake by nerve terminal because Ach does not have uptake by nerve terminal

F	C	Acetylcholine secretion because There are no specific drug that increase Ach secretion yet
F	D	Depletion of acetylcholine storage because There are no specific drug that increase Ach secretion yet
F	E	Increase Ach synthesis because There are no specific drug that increase Ach secretion yet

23. The clinical use of muscarinic agonists include

T	A	in treating glaucoma
F	B	in treating asthma because It can cause asthma because it can cause smooth muscle contraction in bronchi
T	C	in treating heart failure
T	D	in treating constipation
T	E	assist bladder emptying

24. The clinical use of muscarinic antagonists include

T	A	treating urinary incontinence
T	B	in treating asthma
T	C	in treating diarrhea
F	D	treat of glaucoma because muscarinic antagonists not used in treatment of glaucoma because ocular effects are produce only after higher penetration doses. Some drug responses lasting several days when applied directly to the eyes.
F	E	treat of hypertension because Because parasympathetic not involve predominantly like sympathetic.

25. unwanted effects of muscarinic antagonists, such as

T	A	Dry mouth
T	B	Constipation
T	C	Blurred vision
T	D	Near vision is impaired
F	E	Increase fluid secretion because Decrease fluid secretion

26. Urinary retention in elderly men with prostatic enlargement can treated by

T	A	muscarinic antagonists
F	B	muscarinic agonists because Antimuscarinics alone not used for treatment of Urinary retention in elderly men with prostatic enlargement but it can be used such as tolterodine in combination with alpha blockers. They act by decreasing acetylcholine effects on the smooth muscle of the bladder, thus helping control symptoms of an overactive bladder.
F	C	indirect Parasympathomimetic because Muscarinic agonists cannot used because. They act by increasing acetylcholine effects on the smooth muscle of the bladder, thus increase symptoms of an overactive bladder.
T	D	alpha blocker
T	E	antiandorgenic drugs

27. Indirect cholinomimetic drug is;

F	A	d-tubocurarine because it is nicotinic receptors blocker at

		neuromuscular junction
F	B	Atropine because Muscarinic blocker
F	C	Pilocarpine because Muscarinic agonist main that direct cholinomimatic drugs
T	D	physostigmine
T	E	neostigmine

28. Muscarinic receptor activation causes all the following EXCEPT

T	A	stimulation of inositol triphosphate signal transducing mechanism
T	B	activation of potassium channel
T	C	opening of sodium channel
T	D	release of nitric oxide from endothelial cells
F	E	open Ca^{2+} channel because Ca^{2+} channel is not control by Muscarinic receptors

29. Intraocular administration of 1% acetylcholine produces:

T	A	contraction of ciliary muscle.
T	B	reduction of intraocular pressure.
T	C	stimulation of lacrimal secretion.
T	D	transient miosis.
F	E	Transient mydriases because It causes Miosis

30. The preferred cholinergic agonist in post operative urinary retention is:

T	A	bethanechol.
F	B	Arecoline because Used clinically as seconf line in Alzheimer's disease
F	C	acetylcholine because it is not used clinically
T	D	physostigmine
F	E	Atropine because it is cholinolytic drug

31. Which of the following is NOT a clinical feature of acute belladona poisoning?

F	A	copious salivation because Decrease salivation and dried moth is occurred.
T	B	urgency for urination but difficult to urinate
T	C	tachycardia
T	D	delirium
T	E	constipation

32. Abrupt withdrawal of clonidine after chronic use causes:

T	A	rise of the blood pressure
T	B	increase heart rate
F	C	Bronchoconstriction because No effect because main effect of clonidine is centrally
F	D	Constipation because Sympathetic is not predominant effect on GIT
F	E	increase intraocular pressure because On effect of clonidine on eyes

33. The substances produced locally by one group of cells and exert effects on other types of cells in the same regionare,

T	A	Called Autacoids
T	B	Called also local hormones
F	C	Work only on parasympathetic nervous system because It work on any cells in body
T	D	Some of analogue clinically used for prevention
T	E	They act through cell membrane receptors

34. The antagonist drugs which work on autacoids pathway used for treatment of

T	A	Migraine and pain
T	B	Inflammatory
T	C	Asthma
T	D	Vomiting
T	E	Allergic reaction

35. True regarding to histamine

T	A	Is synthesized locally form the amino acid histidine
T	B	Orally inactive
T	C	Receptors are G-protein coupled receptors
T	D	Antihistamine drugs compete on H1 receptor

T	E	Histamine analogue used in treat vertigo in Miniere's disease

36. Serotonin (5-hydroxytryptamine),

T	A	Is localized in the intestines, platelets
T	B	Is Synthesised from the amino acid tryptophan
T	C	Is Metabolised by a monoamine oxidise, adehydrogenase, and decarboxliase
T	D	Has cell membrane receptors belong to G-protein
T	E	In CNS is considered as neurotransmitter

37. True regarding *Eicosanoids*

T	A	Are parts of autacoids mediators
T	B	Include Prostaglandins and Leukotrienes
T	C	Are polyunsaturated essential fatty acids
T	D	Are synthesised by phospholipase A, cyclo-oxygenase (COX) and lipooxyganse
T	E	The half-life of most prostaglandins in the circulation is less than 1 minute.

38. True regarding prostanoids

T	A	Encompasse the prostaglandins and the thromboxanes
T	B	Prostanoid receptors which are typical G-protein-coupled receptors

T	C	Causes bronchoconstriction
T	D	Used in gastric ulcer
F	E	In treatment of allergy because it is one of inflammatory mediators and produce some of allergy symptom.

39. True regarding therapeutic uses of prostanoid analogues

T	A	Termination of pregnancy and induction of labour
T	B	To prevent ulcers associated with NSAD
T	C	Treatment of glaucoma
T	D	To prevent platelet aggregation
F	E	Auto immune disease because Auto immune disease this is disease in which the body's immune system has become hyper-defensive, attacking the cells, organs, and tissues of its own body as if they are diseases that need to be destroyed. prostanoid analogues not reduce this effect.

40. True regarding leukotrienes

T	A	Are synthesised from arachidonic acid by lipoxygenase-catalysed pathways.
T	B	Receptors utilise inositol trisphosphate and increased cytosolic Ca^{2+}
T	C	are potent spasmogens
T	D	cause an increase in mucus secretion
F	E	fall in blood pressure because No effect on blood vessels smooth muscle.

41. True regarding leukotrenes Antagonist

T	A	used in treatment of asthma
T	B	zafirlukast and montelukast are direct leukotrine antagonist.
T	C	Zileuton is indirect of leukotreine blocker
T	D	Important when used for treatment of hypertension
T	E	Zileuton inhibits lipoxygenase enzyme

42. True regarding chemotherapy

T	A	Is designed to inhibit/kill the infecting organism and to have no/minimal effect on the recipient.
F	B	Is designed to inhibit/kill the infecting organism and to have effect on the recipient because The main site of action of chemotherapy agents are organism. And other effects will be considered as a side effect or secondary effects.
T	C	Treatment of systemic infections with specific drugs that selectively suppress the infecting microorganism without significantly affecting the host.
F	D	Treatment of systemic infections with specific drugs that selectively suppress the infecting microorganism without significantly affecting the host because Once drug inter systemic circulation will be distributed in all the body tissues so it will has effects.
	E	

43. General principles of antimicrobial use are:

T	A	It is not to be prescribed indiscriminately.
T	B	Rapidly acting and selective drugs to be used wherever possible
F	C	It is prescribed for any types of infectious conditions because There are several causes of infections such as virus, bacteria and parasites.
T	D	Broad-spectrum are used when a specific one cannot be determined or not suitable.
F	E	It is stopped immediately when symptoms of infection disappear because Should time course should be continue

44.True regarding therapeutic index (TI) of antimicrobials

T	A	penicillins, some cephalosporins and erythromycin have high therapeutic index
T	B	Aminoglycosides, tetracyclines and chloramphenicol have low therapeutic index
F	C	Polymyxin B, vancomycin and amphotericin B have very low therapeutic index because amphotericin B is antifungal drug not antibiotic
T	D	Antibiotic with high TI can be prescribed for pregnant women
F	E	Antibiotic with low TI can be prescribed for pregnant women because It cannot prescribed for pregnant women cause

45.True regarding resistance

T	A	It refers to unresponsiveness of a microorganism to an antimicrobial drugs
T	B	Natural resistance does not pose a significant clinical problem.
F	C	Natural resistance does pose a significant clinical problem because Natural resistance means that the bacteria are 'intrinsically' resistant. For example, Streptomyces has some genes responsible for resistance to its own antibiotic. Other examples include organisms that lack a transport system or a target for the antibiotics. So this type of resistance dose not developed due to used antibiotic in second time so their is no any clinical significant
T	D	Acquired resistance poses a significant clinical problem
F	E	Cross resistance does not pose a significant clinical problem because Acquired resistance refers to bacteria that are usually sensitive to antibiotics, but are liable to develop resistance. Acquired resistance is often caused by mutations in chromosomal genes, or by the acquisition of mobile genetic elements, such as plasmids or transposons, which carry the antibiotic resistance genes. So this type of resistance develop during use antibiotic so it has a significant clinical problem

46. True regarding Prevention of drug resistance

T	A	No indiscriminate and inadequate or unduly prolonged use of AMAs
T	B	Rapidly acting and selective (narrowspectrum) AMAs whenever possible
T	C	Use combination of AMAs whenever prolonged therapy is

		undertake
F	D	Use broad-spectrum drugs because Broad spectrum of drug not necessary that the drug dose not has resistance because resistance will be depend on organism and pharmacokinetics of antibiotics parameters.
F	E	Antimicrobial is prescribed after sensitivity test because Even though if the drug prescribed after sensitivity test will not prevent drug resistance because the organism can mutate and resistance can be developed at any time.

47.True combined use of antimicrobial drugs

T	A	To achieve synergism
F	B	To achieve potency because Achieve potency main reduce the dose. In the combination of antimicrobial drug should the dose not change.
T	C	To reduce severity of adverse effects
T	D	To prevent of resistance
F	E	To broden the spectrum of antimicrobial action because Some antibiotics have broad spectrum so no need to use combination to achieve

48.True regarding failure of antimicrobial therapy

T	A	Improper selection of drug, dose, route or duration of treatment.
T	B	Treatment begun too late
T	C	Failure to take necessary adjuvant measures

T	D	Poor host defence
T	E	Presence of dormant or altered organisms

49. Use the accompanied diagram for the following questions:

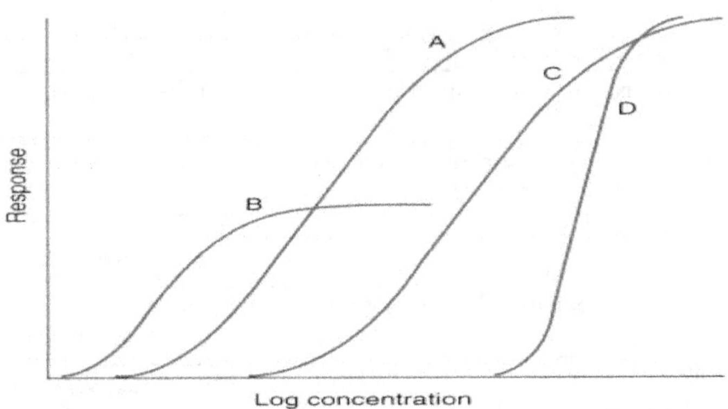

49.1) Which of the following drugs would require the most care when administrating, if the upper portion of the dose-response curve signified severe toxicity?

F	A	Because the therapeutic dose high and the elimination phase is directly proportional to the absorption phase.
T	B	
F	C	The same with A
F	D	The same with A

49.2) Which drug is the least efficacious?

F	A	Drug shows high response main that has high efficiency. So all drugs A, C, and D show high response and false options.
T	B	B

F	C	Drug shows high response main that has high efficiency. So all drugs A, C, and D show high response and false options.
F	D	Drug shows high response main that has high efficiency. So all drugs A, C, and D show high response and false options.

49.3) Intrinsic activity is a drug's ability to elicit:

F	A	Strong receptor binding because They well be based on affinity
F	B	Weak receptor binding because They well be based on affinity
T	C	Response
F	D	Excretion because No relation with intrinsic activity
F	E	Distribution because No relation with intrinsic activity

49.4) Which direction would a partial agonist shift the dose-response curve when compared to a full agonist?

F	A	To the left because Only an agonist because has high efficacy
F	B	To the right because Only competitive antagonist shift the curve response of agonist
F	C	Down because In non0-compatitive antagonist
F	D	Up because Synergistic drug
T	E	To the right and possibly down

49.5) Which direction would a competitive antagonist (plus agonist) shift the dose response curve when compared to a full agonist?

F	A	To the left
T	B	To the right

F	C	Down
F	D	Up
F	E	To the right and possibly down

See the previous MCQ

ABOUT THE AUTHOR

Associate Professor Dr. Redhwan Ahmed Al-Naggar obtained his PhD in community Medicine specialized in Epidemiology from the National University of Malaysia. Then he has obtained cancer prevention and control fellow from USA. He is working in as Associate Professor of Population Health and Preventive Medicine, Faculty of Medicine, Universiti Teknologi MARA (UiTM), Malaysia. He has published more than 156 original articles in refereed journals in more than a dozen journals, three books and produced more than 20 conference papers including international and national conferences. He is currently the Chief-editor of international Medical journals. Academic editor for PLOS, SCIENCEDOMAIN international, British Journal of Education, Society & Behavioural Science and others. Editorial board member for OMICS Group eBooks, Journal Community Medicine and Health Education, Journal of Pharmacy and Nutrition Sciences, Journal of Solid Tumors, Lifescience Global and others. Reviewer of local journals and international impact factor journal such as Asia Pacific journal of public Health, Journal of Peace, Gender and Development studies, Malaysian Journal of Medical Science, BMC Public Health, PLOS one, Vaccine Journal, BMC Research Notes, Journal of Solid Tumors, British Journal of Education, Society & Behavioural Science, BMC Women's Health, Medical Journal of Malaysia and others. In 2010 he was the winner of the best research Award in the Management and Science university, Malaysia which gives to the scientist who have mad outstanding contribution to the field of quantitative and qualitative research. Beside that supervise master and PhD students in community medicine field.

www.ingramcontent.com/pod-product-compliance
Lightning Source LLC
Chambersburg PA
CBHW051332170526
45166CB00002B/779

* 9 7 8 1 4 9 2 2 0 8 2 0 4 *